I0416296

PAA WAH TOKMA
ΦͰͰ ƗͰΤ ϒΦΟΤƐͰ

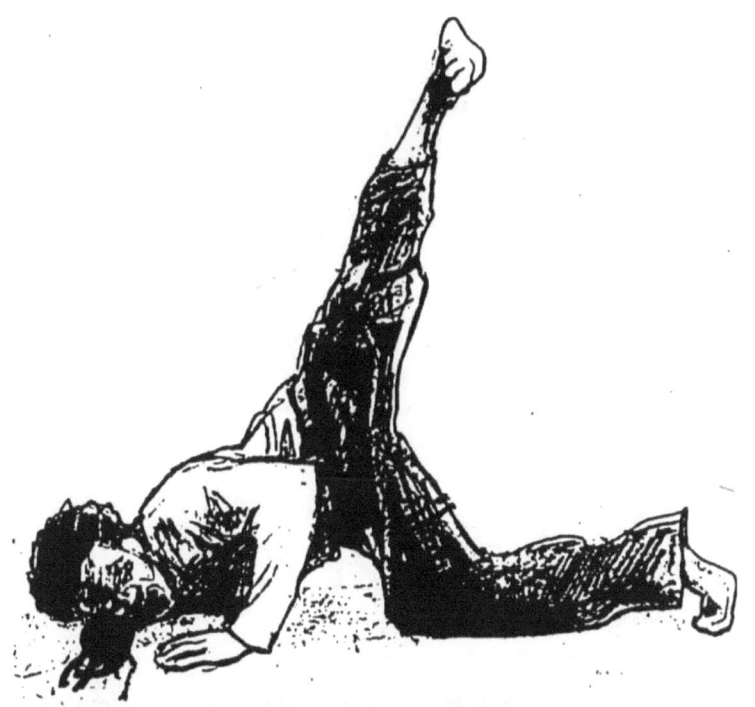

By A'lu Ellis

The First Dance

THE TEMPLE OF KALU UNIVERSAL MARTIAL ARTS PRESENTS:

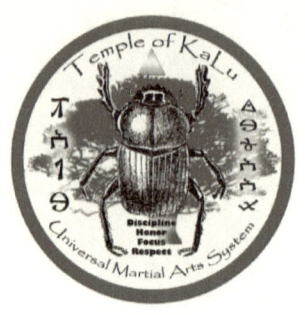

THE FIRST DANCE

Chamber Master A'lu "Wildcat" Ellis

The First Dance

Published by

www.lulu.com

Copyright ©2014 by Ali A. Ellis

Front by A. Bacon

Photographs by A. Bacon

All rights reserved. No part of this book may be reproduced, stored in retrieval system, or transmitted in any form, by any means, including mechanical, electronic, photocopying, recording, or otherwise without prior written permission of the publisher

Printed in the United States of America

ISBN: 978-1-312-35075-5

The First Dance

About The Language

The language that you see utilized in this scroll is called KaLuik. It is a tribal language belonging specifically to the tribe of KaLu. It stems from an ancient Egyptian and African language known then as Meirotic, Napatan, Cuneiform and more recently known as Nuwaupic. This language represents the creation of OUR STUFF and the restoring of our cultural and historical legacy. For more information about the language email thekalucenter@gmail.com.

Peace and Light

ΦϤϤ TⵝↃϤ ϿⵏↃ ЛϤↃJ

The Temple of KaLu Universal Martial Arts

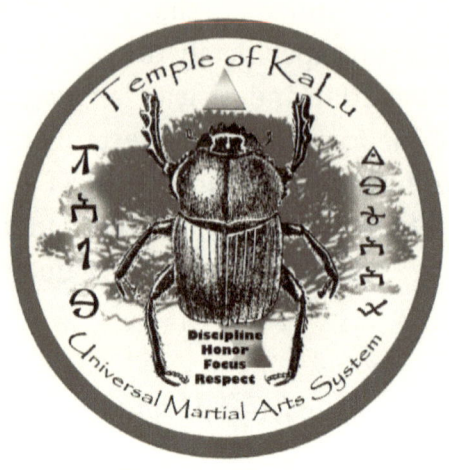

What is The TKUMA? TKUMA is a concept, a principle, a system and a code for the redevelopment and restoration of the true warrior within our communities. It represents the path of the warrior, the mission of the warrior, the duty of the warrior, the skill and the purpose of the warrior. It is a glimpse into the past and the future for the Nubian.

The TKUMA is established as a Temple building program where students within our communities learn the arts but at the same time participate in developmental projects that will erect a true temple within our community. TKUMA is established as a 19 Chamber structure with each chamber containing the principles of various fighting styles mastered by members of our community. Each Chamber allows the student to get nearer to the 19th seat which will symbolize the mastery of TKUMA.

The First Dance

ach community master will have an honorary seat within the temple n order to share their skill set. Students will learn principles of Zarate, Kung Fu, Tae Kwon Do, Capoieria, Jeet Kun Do, Jujitsu, Aikido and other styles as well as ancients styles dating from the birthplace of all martial arts, NUBIA (Tama Re, Khemet, Africa, Alkebulan, etc.)

Students will advance by way of sashes and keys. Each key represents a point within a Chamber that they will master such as focus, discipline, skill, etc. Sashes will be awarded at various intervals in the Chamber advancement.

TKUMA is not meant to be the only martial arts structure in the community. It is only meant as a developmental tool that all other schools can benefit from as well as assist in creating an inter-communal union of martial artists that we are responsible for without interference from outside of our community.

These scrolls are meant to be an introduction into the basics of the TKUMA. Each Chamber URA (Master) will have the opportunity to pen a scroll within the TKUMA system. This is all in the vein of creating OUR STUFF.

Peace and light

URA Karaam (Black Owl) Ellis-El
SKS Black Belt
Founder of TTKUMA

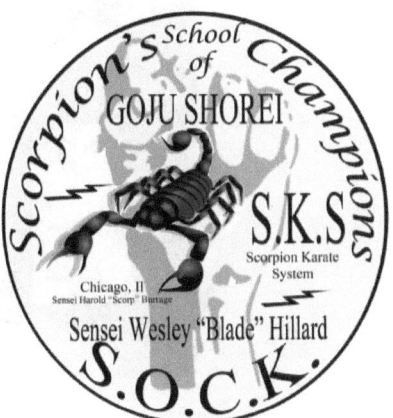

The Author
Chamber Master A'lu "Wildcat" Ellis

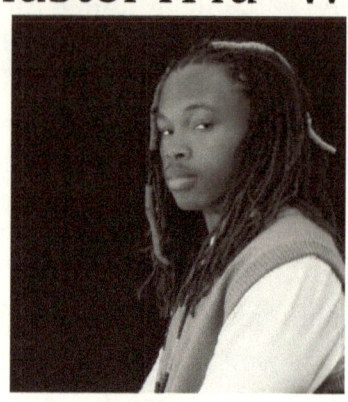

Contributor
Chamber Master & Founder URA
Karaam "Black Owl" Ellis-El

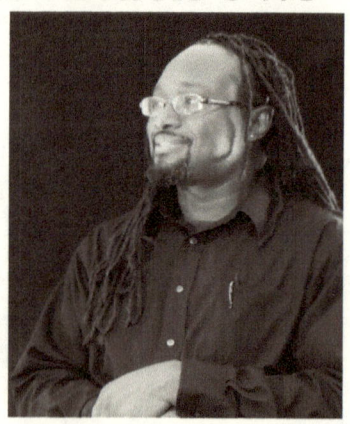

ΦƐƐ ŦƐT ʌ⊕ʎƷƐ

The First Dance

BASICS

BREATH

Proper breathing is crucial to good martial arts. If you don't not breathe properly, your moves will lack full power and you will lack stamina. Good breathing oxygenates the body and helps avoid cramps and unnecessary muscular strain and tension.

Whenever you breathe in, imagine that you are pushing the oxygen down into your stomach. Your abdomen should extend. Then as you exhale, envision the air rising from your abdomen up into your chest, through your neck, and finally out of your mouth. Your abdomen should flatten on the exhalation. Breathe in through your nose and out of your mouth.

MAKING A PROPER FIST

Hold your hand open. Keeping your thumb as it is, curl your fingers tightly into the palm of your hand. Then lay your thumb down over your index and middle fingers.

STRETCHING

The First Dance

Before doing any physical activities, it is good to stretch your body thoroughly. It warms and loosens the muscles, and calms the mind allowing you to more easily perform the dance. Stretching also helps prevent soreness. Breathing is absolutely essential to proper stretching, so never forget to incorporate it at all times.

RELAXATION

The mind and body of the true Martial Arts practitioner is always calm and relaxed. Being at ease helps improve focus, perception, reaction time, and overall performance. When perfoming Paa Wah Tokma try not to tense up or focus on anything other than the movements and the breath.

The First Dance

The following information was written and or researched and documented from an unknown author who I would like to give credit to and given to us by our Grandfather Sensei Harold Scorpion Burrage

HISTORY AND DEVELOPMENT OF KARATE

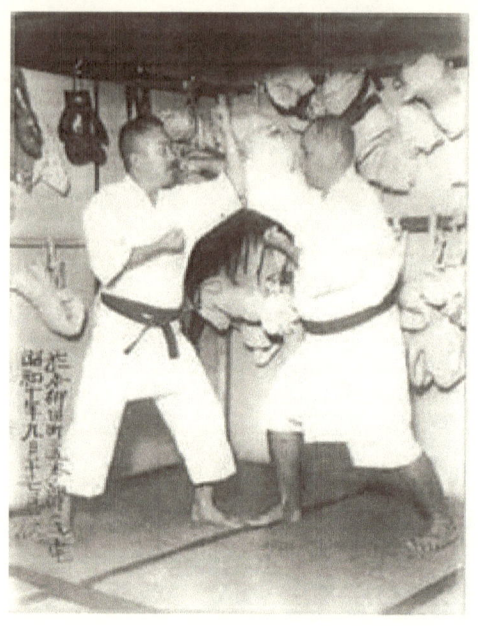

Karate is a form of Martial Art which dates back over fourteen hundred years to about 520 AD. There are no volumes of books to research its history, and the word of mouth information has been comprised by secrecy and the secret societies often associated with Karate. In addition, there have been some inconsistencies due to translation of oriental languages into English. The original art form or styles, fortunately, and in some cases unfortunately, have been modified over time by different groups in their attempts to customize Karate to their own needs and capabilities.

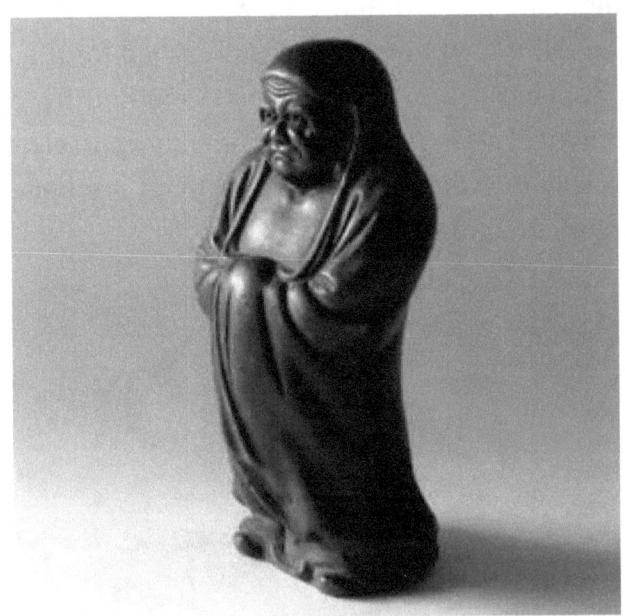

DARUMA BODHIDHARMA, a native of Conjeevaram (near Madras, a state in southeastern India, populated mostly by Dravidians, a people of African Ancestry), left India around 520 AD enroute to China to teach Buddhism. He was also the founder of Zen Buddhism.

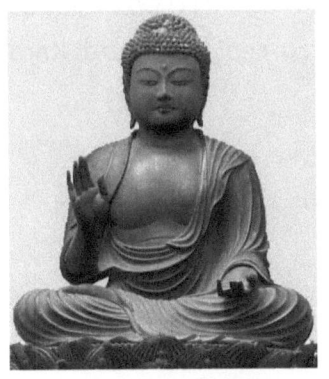

The First Dance

While teaching his followers in the Shaolin Temple (In the Hunan Province of China), he noticed that they were in poor condition. He said to them: "Although the way of Buddha is preached for the soul, the body and soul are inseparable..." "I shall give a method by which you can develop your physical strength enough to enable yourselves to attain the essence of the way of Buddha." These teachings are believed to be the earliest beginnings of Karate.

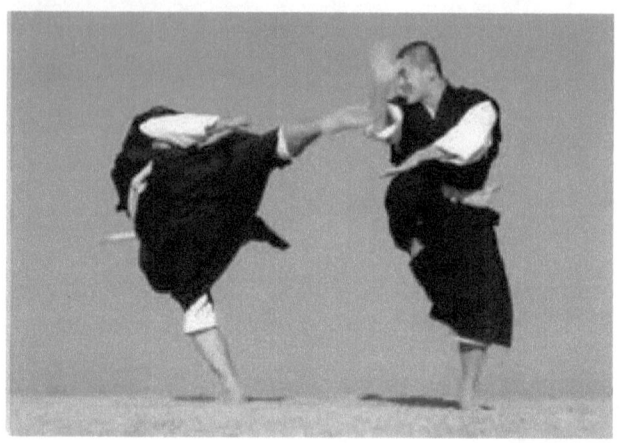

As many years went by, these original methods became known as SHOREIN-JI KENPO (named for the area it evolve in). Eventually this Martial Art form reached the RYUKYU Islands off the coast of Japan. Further development occurred here and Karate at that time became known as OKINAWA-TE.

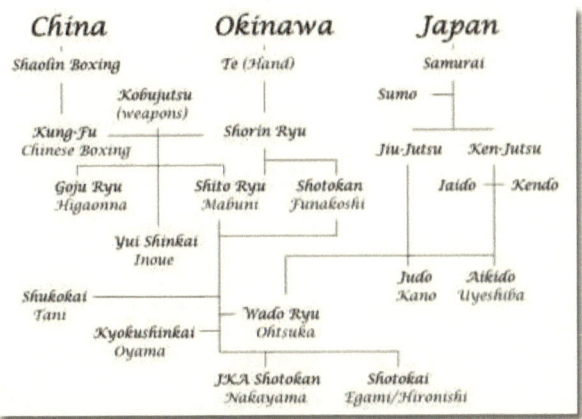

China | Okinawa | Japan

Shaolin Boxing — Te (Hand) — Samurai
Kobujutsu (weapons)
Kung-Fu Chinese Boxing — Shorin Ryu — Sumo
Jiu-Jutsu — Ken-Jutsu
Goju Ryu Higaonna — Shito Ryu Mabuni — Shotokan Funakoshi — Iaido — Kendo
Yui Shinkai Inoue
Shukokai Tani
Kyokushinkai Oyama — Wado Ryu Ohtsuka
Judo Kano — Aikido Uyeshiba
JKA Shotokan Nakayama — Shotokai Egami/Hironishi

During the early 17th century in Okinawa, possession of any weapon by the common people was strictly forbidden. In 1609 the government of Japan confiscated all weapons. In order for the people to protect themselves from bandits and oppressors, they had to learn and perfect unarmed (empty-hand) self-defense techniques. They also developed various weapons techniques with their available farm tools. These techniques were the earlier forms of our present day empty hand and weapon katas. Because of this great need, this Okinawan Martial Arts form continued to advance. Over the next 300 hundred years there was continuous exchange between China and Okinawa resulting in the current styles of Karate we practice.

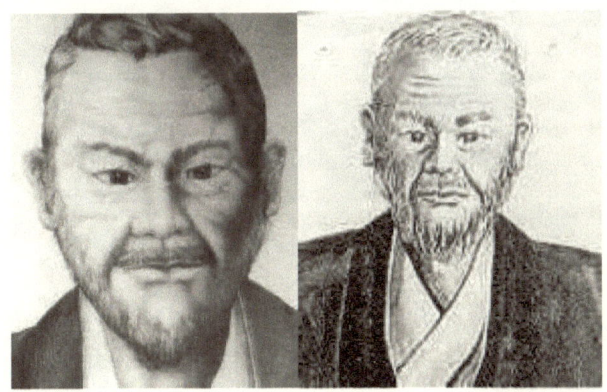

The First Dance

Masters Azato and Itosu

Masters Azato and Itosu were the teachers who instructed GICHIN FUNAKOSHI, the so-called founder of modern day Karate. This distinction is given to him because of his tremendous contributions, including historical documentation, promoting Karate and formalizing so much of what we do today. This includes various exercises, the 19 or so standard katas, sparring techniques and the different promotional or ranking classification ie., DAN and KYU. Master Funakoshi was born in Shura, Okinawa in 1868 and died in Tokyo, Japan in 1957. The first dojo which he founded was called SHOTOKAN and opened in Japan in the spring of 1936.

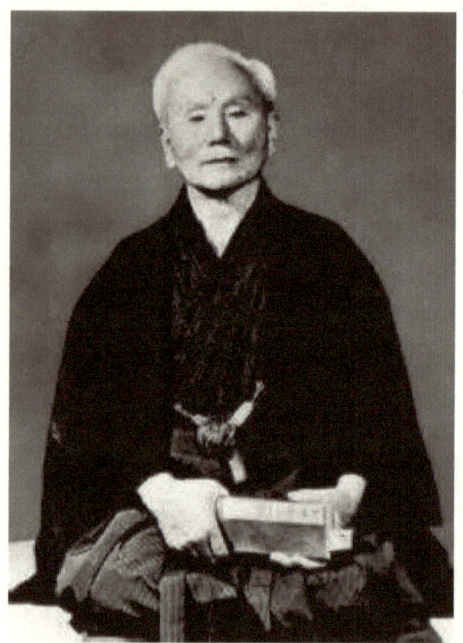

GICHIN-FUNAKOSHI

He is the author of many books, most notable, Karate Do, My Way Of Life, and Karate Kyohan from which a great deal of information in this manual was derived. Additional research was obtained from the heart of Karate Do by Shigeru Egami in Karate's History and Tradition by Bruce A. Haines.

In 1902 Karate broke its centuries old secrecy when for the first time it was introduced to the general public in a public high school in Okinawa, as part of the physical education of the high school students. Master Funakoshi continued his promotion of Karate and in 1916 or 1917 authorized the first demonstration of Karate outside of Okinawa in Kyoto, Japan. At that time this was the official center of all Martial Arts. During World War II, American soldiers stationed in Okinawa and Japan were introduced to Karate, thus American Karate has a history of about 70 years.

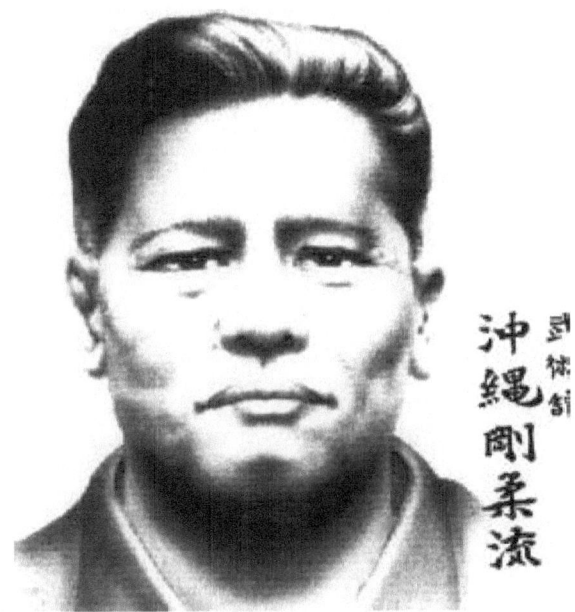

Shojun Miyagi, a student of Master Funakoshi, who taught at the Kyoto Imperial University introduced a style of Karate known as GOJU. GOJU means 50 in Japanese and therefore implies that there at least 50

diversified hard and soft styles. Our style is called GOJU SHOREI and is a direct descendant from this original system. In addition, we say that our style employs a hard and low stance.

Tradition says that in the old days a Martial Artist started to train and kept his pants secure by the use of a white belt. As he continued to train and with the passage of time, his belt gradually turned dark in color until it was finally black. At that time, he wore a black belt. Today a black belt means that the wearer has trained for several years and has gradually reached the high and honorable rank of "black belt". In GOJU SHOREI a beginner wears a white belt. After a period of learning the student is gradually promoted to yellow, orange, blue, gree, purple, brown 3rd degree, brown 2nd degree, brown 1st degree, and finally black belt. Some would say that now your study of Karate can really begin... Certainly you should be refining your information, skills and getting into the deeper meaning of Karate. Black Belt or DAN classification has 10 degrees, the first degree is the lowest, and the 10th is the highest. Those students holding rank from yellow to brown belts, can promote other students, however it is not official until they have received recognition from a black belt.

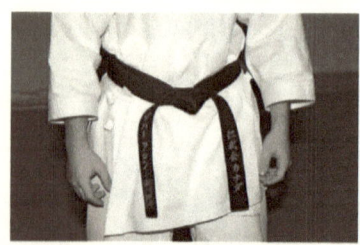

A quick review of Karate's history reveals origins in India, then China, Okinawa, Japan, and other parts of the world. It had religious beginnings, ie., Zen Buddhism, and several name changes, to include KENPO or SHORENJI KENPO, OKINAWA-TE and finally Karate. Kara translates as

The First Dance

"empty"; Te translates as "hand", hence KARATE. The definition of Karate is the art or science of empty hand fighting using various parts of the body such as hands, feet, elbow, etc.

The public thinks of Karate as breaking boards, tile crushing with the fists and head, brick breaking, etc. Such demonstrations or techniques are sometimes used demonstrate the power of Karate. These feats are only done to show the strength of the fists, forearm elbow, or foot and by itself has nothing to do with the true art and purpose of the Karate.

A common feature of Karate is speed and one's ability to properly strike the vulnerable or vital areas of an attacker's body. Not all movements and techniques are deadly to an antagonist. A well trained Karate Ka (student or practitioner) can inflict the amount of damage he desires. Just enough damage to stop the attack without permanently injuring his adversary. Importantly, this ability also protects one against breaking the law by using excessive force. One quickly realizes that you do not need to be a large or exceptionally strong individual in order to defend yourself. Rather, the reason the Martial Artist is victorious is usually because of knowledge and speed.

In addition to the discipline, self confidence and esteem you get from the study of Karate, it is great exercise. The practice of Karate uses all parts of the body, thereby helping you stay in good physical condition. You will find that engaging in Karate training is exciting and rewarding. Anyone can participate, male or female, young or old according to your own desires and capabilities.

The First Dance

Katakana (カタカナ)

wa	ra	ya	ma	pa	ba	ha	na	da	ta	za	sa	ga	ka	a
ワ	ラ	ヤ	マ	バ	バ	ハ	ナ	ダ	タ	ザ	サ	ガ	カ	ア
	ri		mi	pi	bi	hi	ni	di	chi	ji	shi	gi	ki	i
	リ		ミ	ピ	ビ	ヒ	ニ	ヂ	チ	ジ	シ	ギ	キ	イ
	ru	yu	mu	pu	bu	fu	nu	du	tsu	zu	su	gu	ku	u
	ル	ユ	ム	プ	ブ	フ	ヌ	ヅ	ツ	ズ	ス	グ	ク	ウ
	re		me	pe	be	he	ne	de	te	ze	se	ge	ke	e
	レ		メ	ペ	ベ	ヘ	ネ	デ	テ	ゼ	セ	ゲ	ケ	エ
n	(o)	ro	yo	mo	po	bo	ho	no	do	to	zo	so	go	ko	o
ン	ヲ	ロ	ヨ	モ	ポ	ボ	ホ	ノ	ド	ト	ゾ	ソ	ゴ	コ	オ

Finally, a word about Japanese terminology. In Japan, the writter characters do not resemble the English Alphabet. Translation into the English language is done phoenetically and often times with great difficulty. Those reading this manual should know that, rigorous effort has been made to correctly translate the Japanese into English. There are some terms that have been past down for many years and widely accepted, therefore somewhat resistant to change. Where these inconsistencies may exist, we respectfully apologize.

SEVEN PRINCIPLES OF GOJU SHOREI KARATE

1. KARATE, in all of its aspects, begins with and ends with courtesy and respect
2. You must be totally serious. Your training and attitude will determine your ability to perform.
3. Train vigorously with your heart and soul, so that your mind and body become one. In this way, what you learn will be remembered always.
4. Do not become complacent...Always remain a student...By doing so, you will continue to learn.
5. Avoid flattery, conceit, dogmatism, and conflict.
6. Be humble but confident. See yourself as you really are. Strive to adopt what is truly meritorious in others.

7. Abide with honor, respect, strength, courage, and the rule of ethics in your daily life.

OUR MOTTO

A well trained body, a well-trained mind, and a focused spirit are keys to becoming a master.

OUR CREED

The Scorpion system of karate trains teachers, not students.

THREE DEGREES OF POWER

HARD, MEDIUM HARD, SOFT

FIVE DEGREES OF FOCUS

1. Not to touch
2. Come within an inch
3. Touch lightly
4. Touch to injure
5. Touch to kill

SEVEN VITAL AND FATAL SPOTS

1. Top of the head
2. Temple
3. Nasal area
4. Larynx
5. Solar Plexus
6. Seika Tanden
7. The Groin

TYPES OF HAND POSITIONS

1. CLOSED HAND STRIKE

    to stop or hurt someone

2. OPEN HAND STRIKE

    for quickness or to reroute or deflect, where deflection means to turn from a straight or fixed course.

COLOR OF BELTS

1.	WHITE	SHYROHI
2.	YELLOW	KIRYUE
3.	ORANGE	SICHIKYU
4.	BLUE	GOKYU
5.	GREEN	YONKYU
6.	PURPLE	ROKKYU
7.	BROWN	EQUE-1ST DEGREE BROWN

NEQUE-2ND DEGREE BROWN

SANQUE -3RD DEGREEE BROWN

BROWN – CHAH EE ROH EE

BLACK – KOO ROH OHBEE

QUE = Boy   DAN =Man

8. SHOEDAN – 1ST DEGREE

NIDAN – 2ND DEGREE

SANDAN – 3RD DEGREE

YODAN – 4TH DEGREE

The First Dance

GODAN – 5TH DEGREE
ROKUDAN – 6TH DEGREE
SICHIDAN – 7TH DEGREE
HACHIDAN 8TH DEGREE
KUDAN 9TH DEGREE
JUDAN 10TH DEGREE

PAA WAH TOKMA

The Martial Arts forms, katas, shoreis, etc are called "dances" in The Temple of KaLu Universal Martial Arts. Paa Wah Tokma translates in English as "The First Dance". It is the first of a series of dances that will be mastered in each chamber. Each dance will reflect the principles of that chamber.

THE FIRST CHAMBER

Paa Wah Tokma is based on the Martial Arts principles of Go-ju Shorei Karate, which originates in Okinawa, Japan. Paa Wah Tokma uses the system of Go-ju Shorei called SKS (Scorpion Karate System)-Hard Style, Closed fist founded by Grandfather Sensei Harold "Scorpion" Burrage, as it was taught by my Sensei Blade Hillard.

"KARA" translates as "empty" and "TE" translates as "hand", henceforth "KARATE" translates as "Empty Hand". "DO" translates as "Way", thus "KARATE DO" translates as "Empty Hand Way". The "GOJU" in GOJU SHOREI translates as "50" as in 50 percent hands and 50 percent feet.

Note: In essence the empty hand and the body itself becomes the weapon without weapons

The First Dance

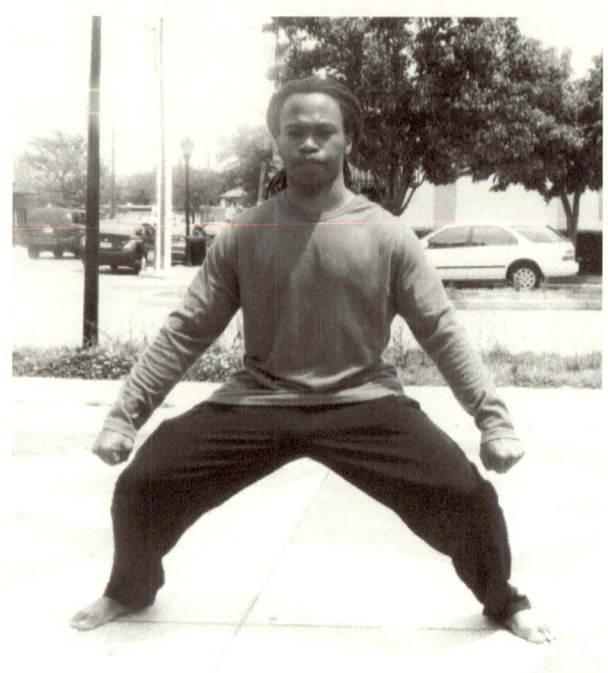

ᏁᎿᎩᏓᏄᎫᏁ ᎫᎬᎩᏌᎨᎪ

NAYISUN GA'YUSHT

HORSE STANCE

Begin all dances with this stance. It is called the "Horse Stance" because it resembles how it looks when someone is riding a horse.

Take a deep breath. Envision your NASHUT (energy) building up in your solar plexus. Ball up your fists. Place your arms in an "X" formation across your chest. Split the "X" and throw arms out to both sides as if blocking both thighs. At the same time, step your right foot out, bending both knees to a bent legged position. Simultaneously release the NASHUT that you built up by yelling "KIA!" (meaning: "spirits meeting") This builds up force and power when performing moves and makes them more effective.

When doing the Horse Stance properly, you should feel a burning sensation in your thighs. The back should be straight. The knees should be bent. The gaze should be directed towards the enemy in front of you. The Horse Stance is not intended for use in an actual fight, rather it is used when performing most martial arts forms.

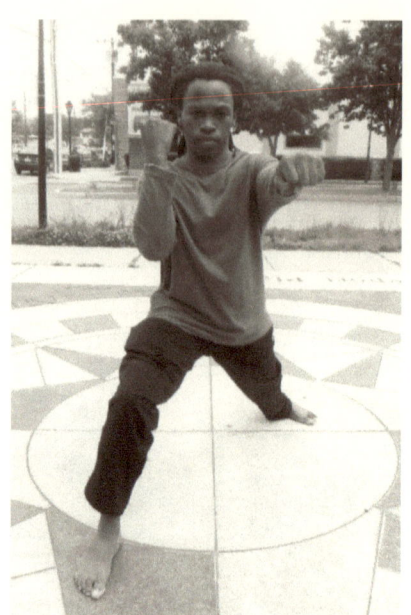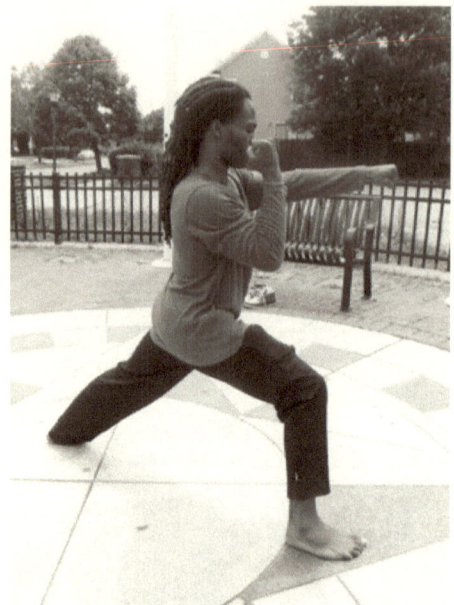

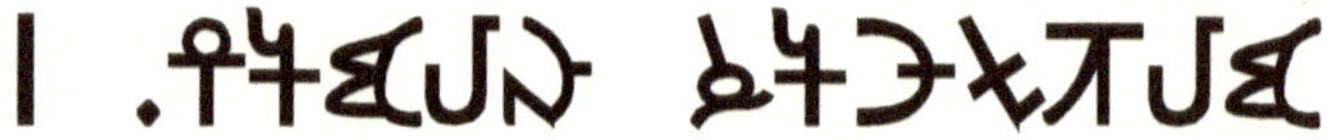

I .ᑭ�538Ո≀ ᑲᒻᒡᕐᄀᒎᒐ I

YAMUN BAGEKUM

RIGHT ZEN PUNCH

From NAYISUN GA'YUSHT, slide your right foot straight forward then to the right, like you are drawing an "L" with your foot. At the same time, form a middle block with your right arm and a straight punch with your left arm.

The First Dance

f done properly, you should not be able to see your toes when looking down at your bent knee. The left leg should be in a slant behind you. Your gaze should be straight ahead.

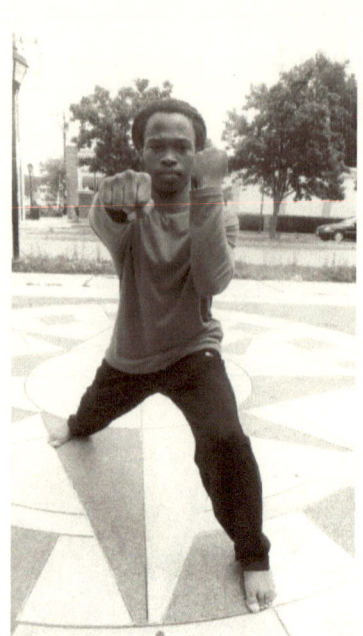 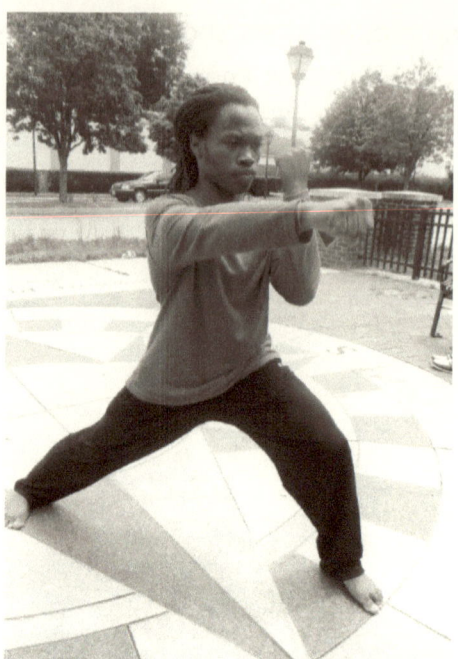

Λ. የ⁴Կ⌐ዓ ኔ⁴Ͻጐ⁷ﬁЈ&

YASUR BAGEKUM

LEFT ZEN PUNCH

Step forward with your left foot, mirroring the last move (YAMUN BAGEKUM) except now it's on your left side.

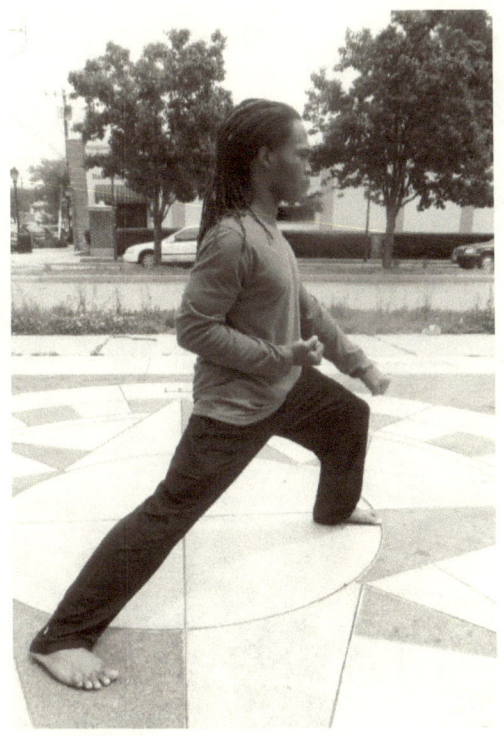

ㅅ. ዋ쑤ᄉᏱ 가ᄀᏌᎦᎫ

YASUR KHAKUNU

LEFT LUNGE STANCE

Keeping your lower body as it was in YASUR BAGEKUM, chamber your right arm and place your left arm over your left leg forming a low block.

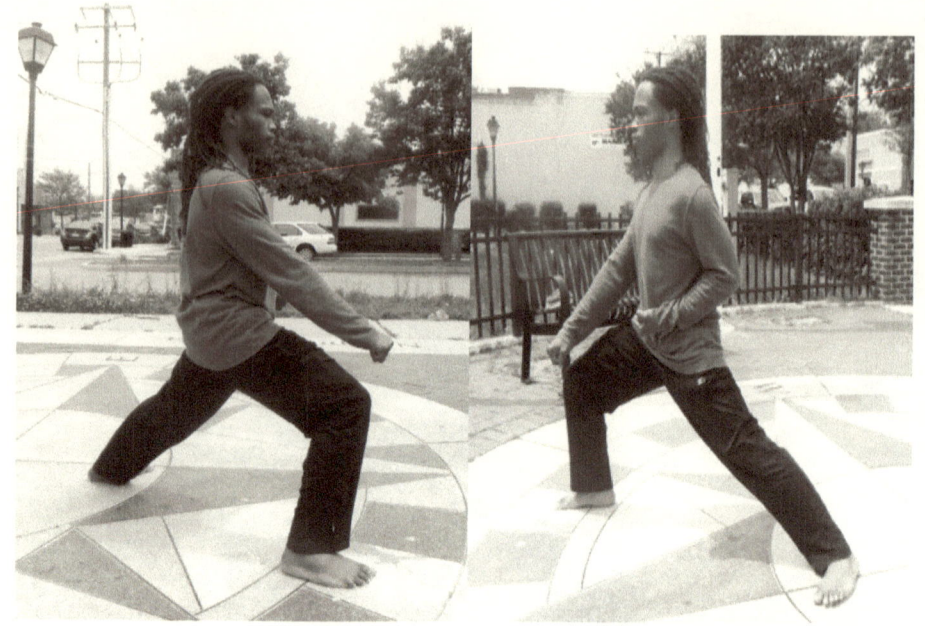

┼. የᎩᏋᎫᎦ ᛏᎩᎯᎫᏅᎫ

YAMUN KHAKUNU

RIGHT LUNG STANCE

Now slide your right foot straight forward then to the right, like you are drawing an "L" with your foot. Chamber your left arm and place your right arm over your right leg forming a low block.

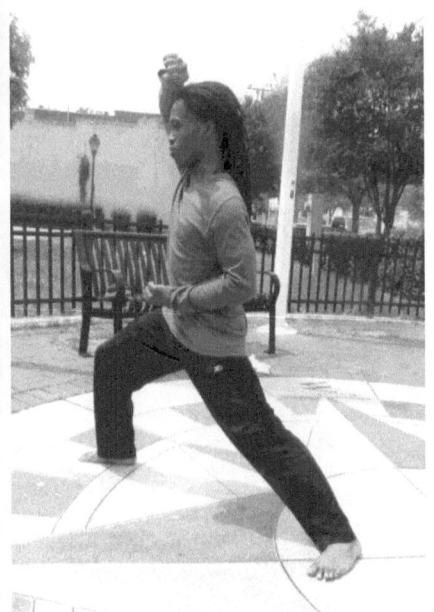 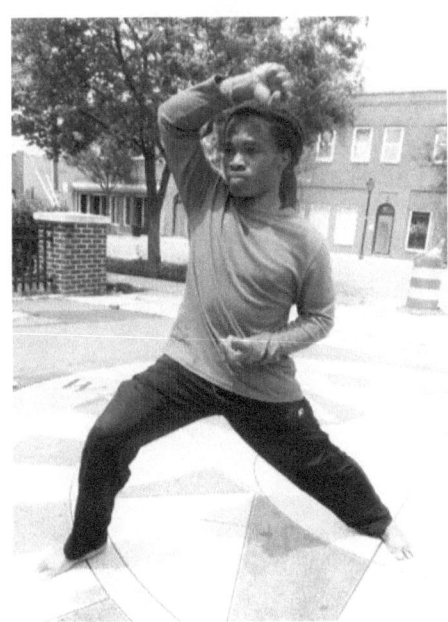

€√ ƆⱡↃ×Ⴕ

A'L GETA

HIGH BLOCK

Keeping your lower body as it was in YAMUN KHAKUNU and your left arm chambered, move your right arm over your head to high block position.

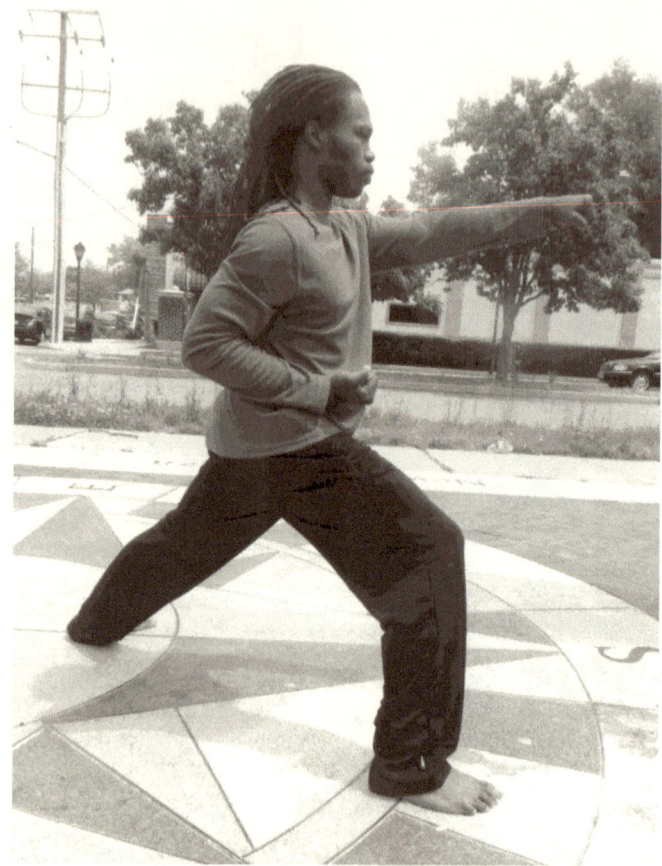

৭৭Чᒍᑫ √ᒋ⊼ᒍᵹ

YASUR LAKUM

LEFT STRIKE

Without moving your lower body, chamber your right arm and straight punch with your left arm.

ⵌ. ᛎ⵲ᛣⵡᛖ ᛖ⵲ᛤⵡᛁ — ᛖ⵲ⵉⵡⵏ ⴼⵌᛐⵈᛐ √⵲ⵊⵡⵉ

YASUR RAFUS – YAMUN ZADUJ LAKUM

LEFT KICK – RIGHT DOUBLE STRIKE

Keeping your arms in the same position as YASUR LAKUM, throw a forward snap kick with your left leg landing into a YAMUN ZADUJ LAKUM. Your left knee is bent, your right leg is in a slant behind you. Chamber your left arm and throw a straight punch with your right arm. Then chamber your right arm and throw a straight left punch.

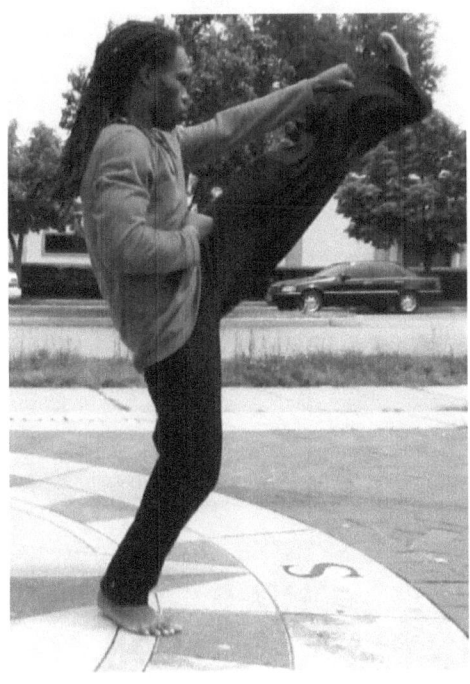

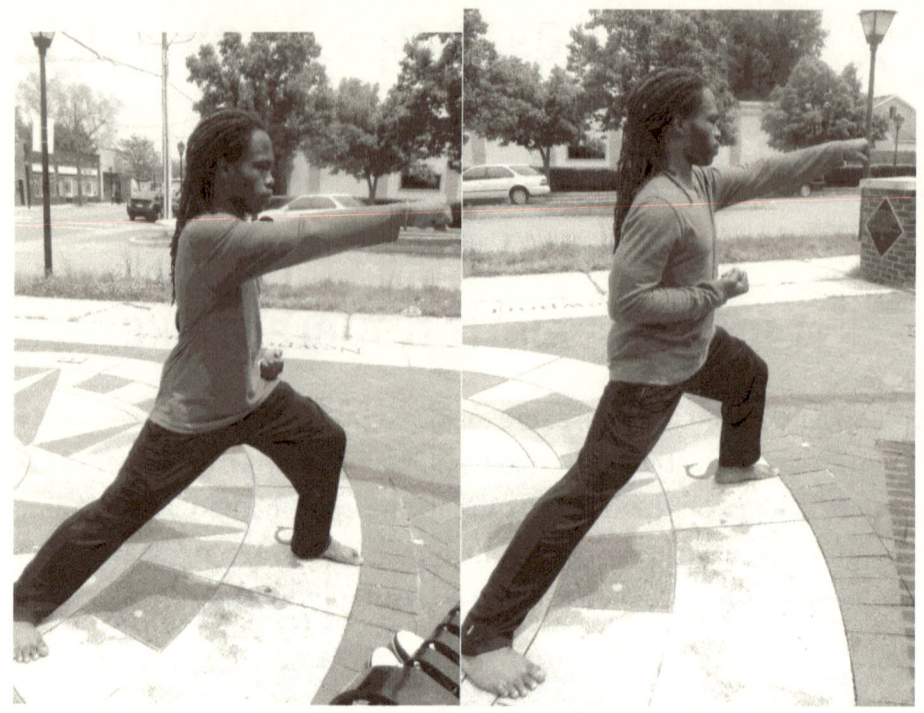

YAMUN ZADUJ LAKUM

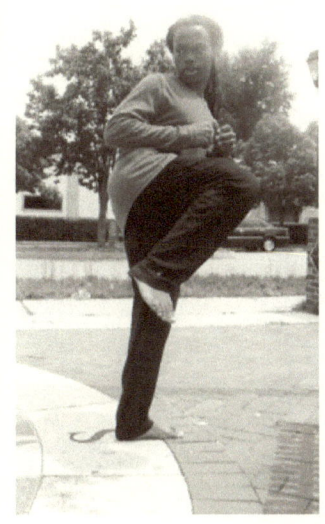 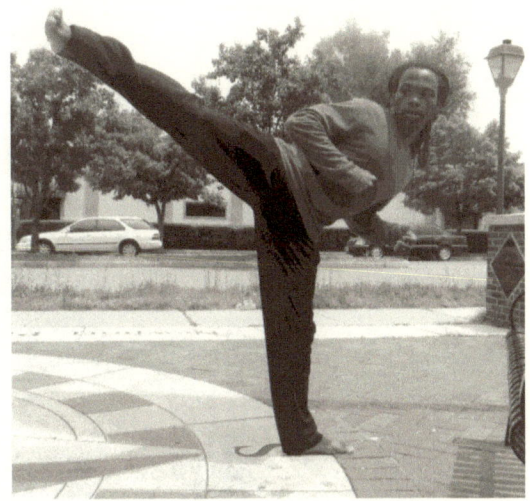

ⵝ. ⵚⵟⵅⵏⵒ ⵟⵟⵣⵟⵗⵍ ⵣⵟ ⵎⵍⵒⵚⵟ

SATHUB HAWALI WA FIBAH

TURN AROUND AND SIDE KICK

Turn your head and look behind you. Chamber your right leg and throw a side kick.   Be sure to kick with the ball of your foot.

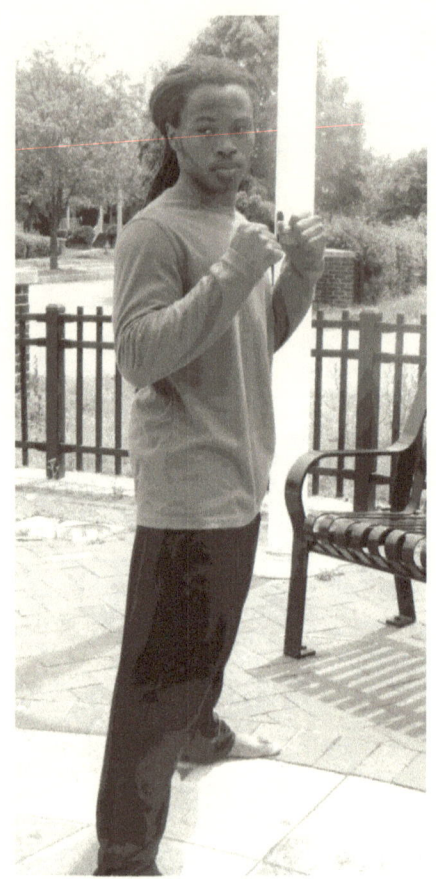

✳. Tⵜⵜⵇⵀⵎⵃ Ɜ€ⵟⵓⵝⵌ

7. HAARUB GA'YUSHT

FIGHTING STANCE

Looking in the same direction, take fighting stance. Bring both your fists up near your chest, while looking at your opponent.

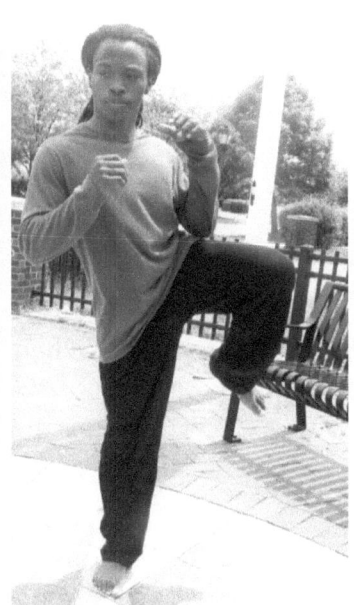

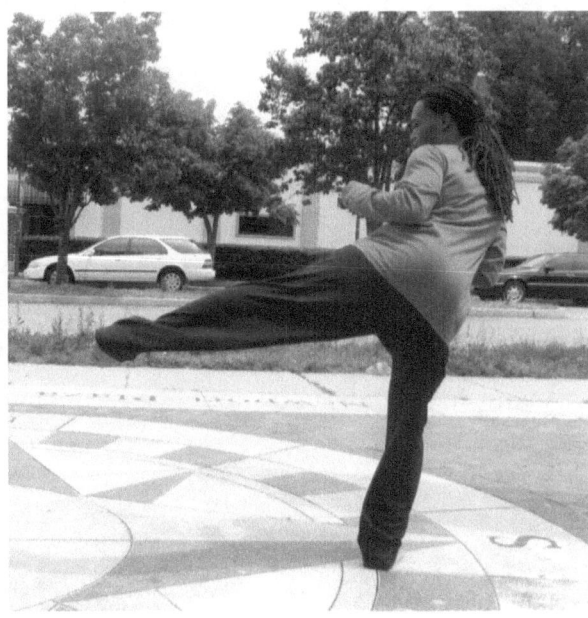

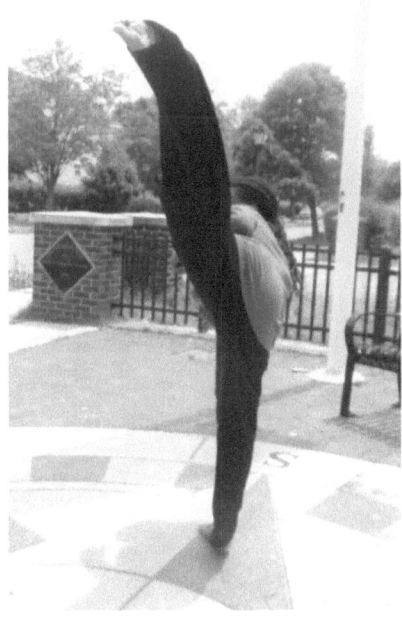

✳. ᚠᛌᛊᛣᛁᚸ ᛏᛌᛘᛣᛠ ⊥√ᛌ ᚱᛣ ᚸᛌᛘᛣᛝ

8. YASUR KHAFUD ILA A'L RAFUS

LEFT LOW TO HIGH KICK

Chamber your left leg, and throw a low – high round house kick. When your foot lands, you should be facing in the opposite direction.

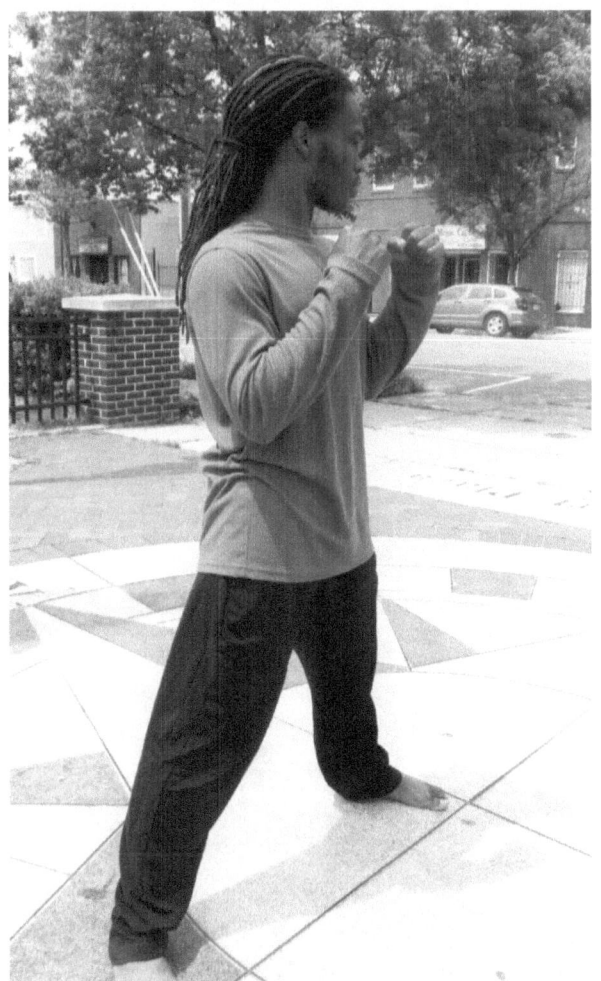

⊛. ꓔꓵꓵꟼꓴꗱ ꓱꗤꝑꓴꝪꓥ

HAARUB GA'YUSHT

FIGHTING STANCE

Take fighting stance by bringing your fists up to your chest.

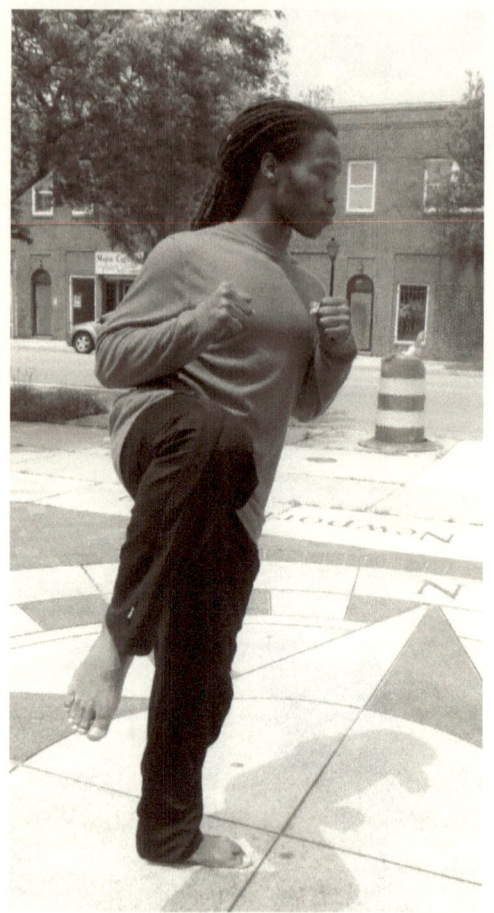

IО. ЄᲤᲣᏏ ᴴᏍᏌᎵᏋᏕ

10. A'YUB WUJEDA

ENEMY FOUND

Keep your hands as they are. Chamber your right leg in preparation for a spin kick.

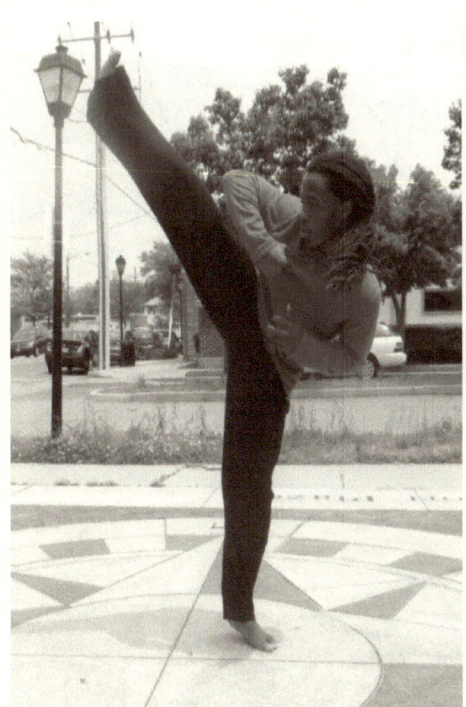 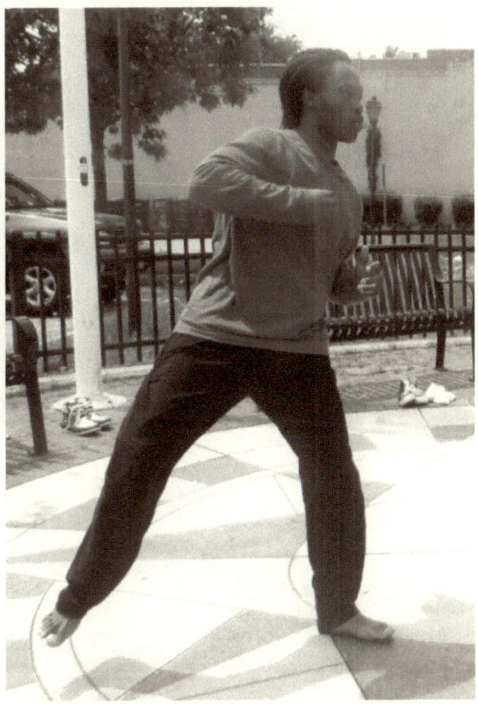

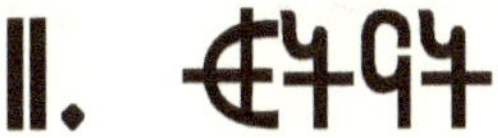

11. Ꮛ�4��

11. GHARA

SPINNING KICK

Look behind you. Throw a spin kick.

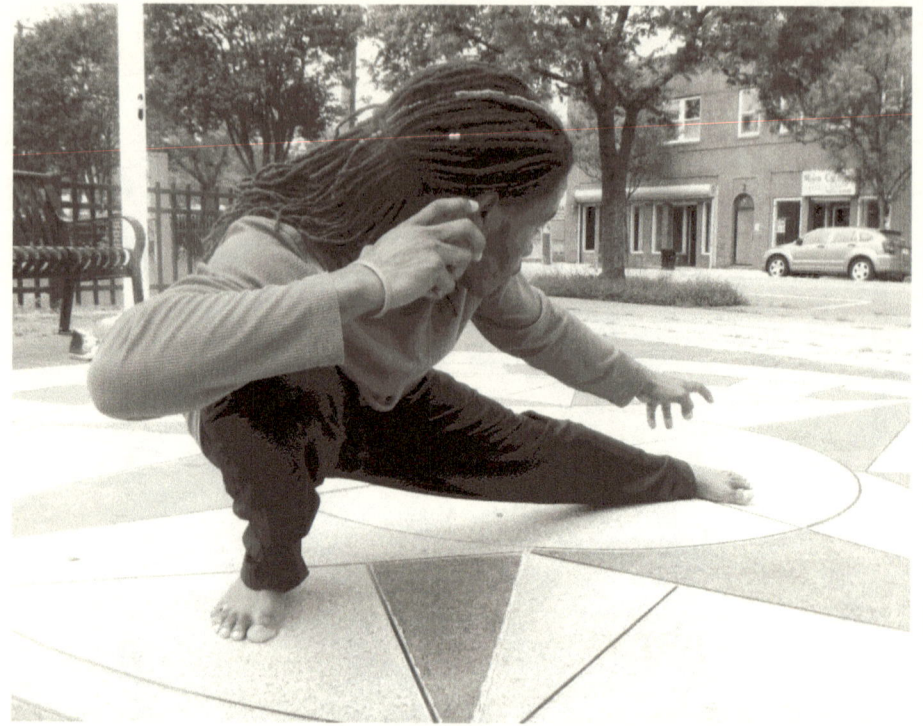

IΛ. ⱵϤT⅂ᘓᒐᓀ ϽᘓᎮᑌƷϪ

12. WAHAMUR GA'YUSHT

CROUCHING STANCE

From the spin kick (GHARA) bend your right leg, dropping all the way to the ground. Place all of your weight on your bent right leg while fully extending your left leg forward. Your buttocks should be right above the ground. Using your arms, mimic the position of your legs, by bending your right arm and extended your left arm. Your hands should resemble eagle's claws.

The First Dance

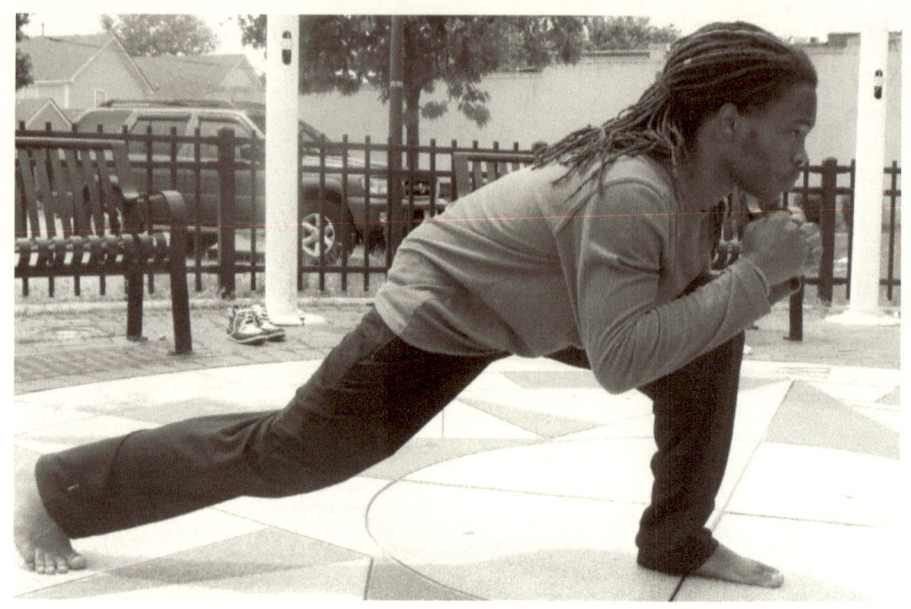

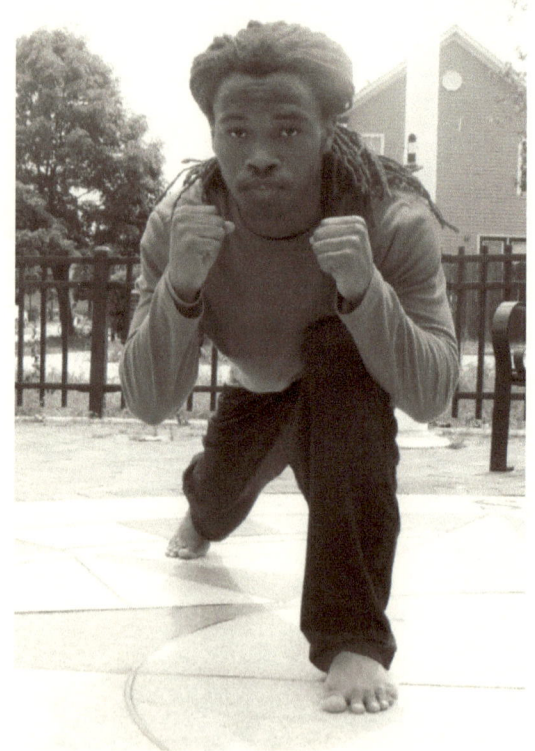

ΙΛ. Ϟ૯Ϟ૯Ϟ ΤϞѫJΛ ΤϞ⅄JϽJ

13. AMAMA KHAFUD KHAKUNU

FORWARD LOW LUNGE STANCE

Quickly, come forward over your left bent knee. Face forward and bring your fists up near your chest. Your right leg should extend behind you with right knee slightly bent.

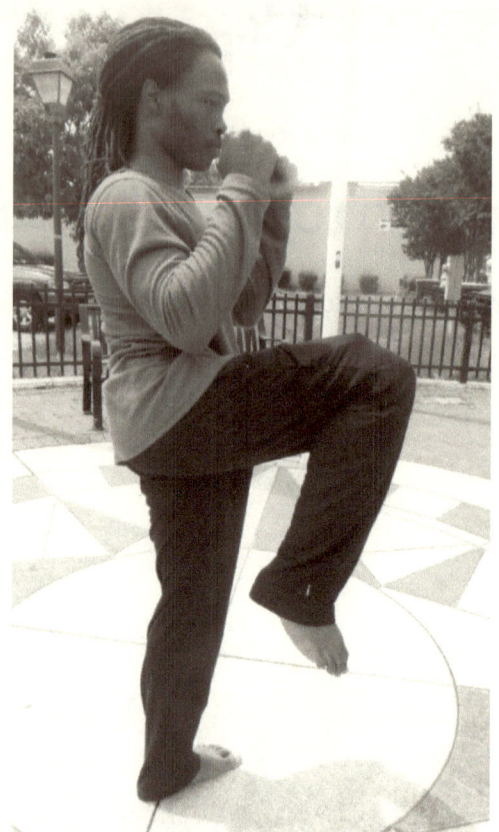

Ⴙ. Ɛ√ ႖ႱᴛႱ♭

14. A'L RUKUB

HIGH KNEE

Keeping your fist up, come to standing high knee with your right leg.

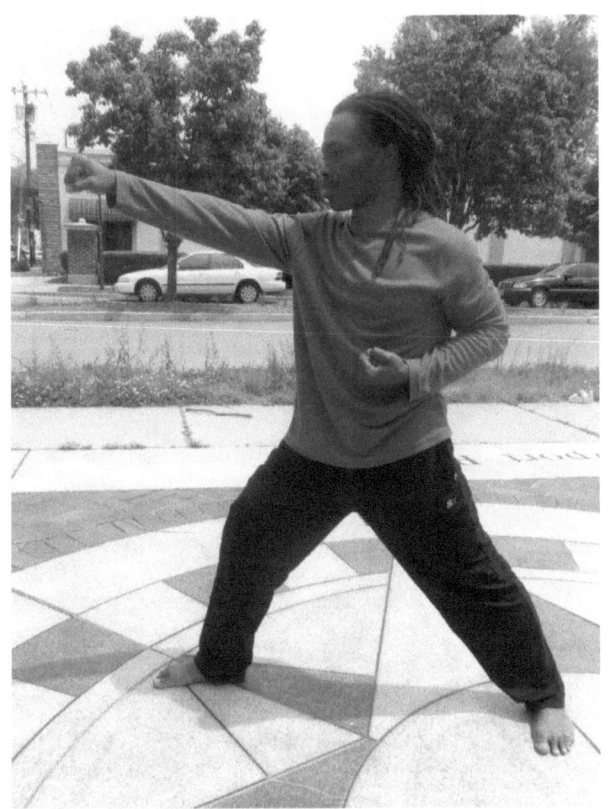

IX. ዋዓᏆᏌᎷ ᎡዓᎯᏌᎯᎫ ᏉዓᎯᏌᏓ

15. YAMUN KHAKUNU LAKUM

RIGHT LUNGE STRIKE

From the high knee, bring your right leg down in front of you. Chamber your left arm and throw a straight forward punch with your right arm.

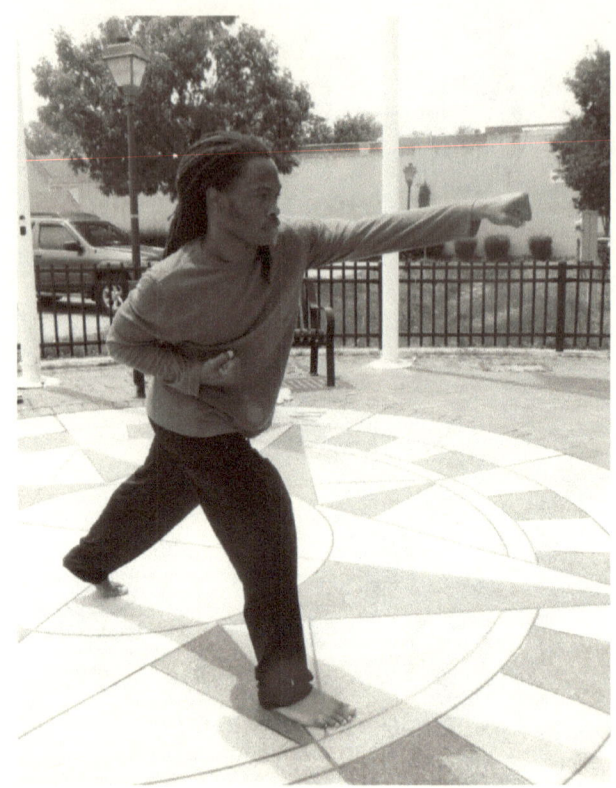

ΙΧ. ΛЧᚻႫႱ‡ √ЧᚒႱƐ

16. DAFUW LAKUM

PUSH STRIKE

Now, chamber your right arm and throw a lunge punch with your left arm. A lunge punch is properly executed by putting your shoulder into the punch and leaning into it.

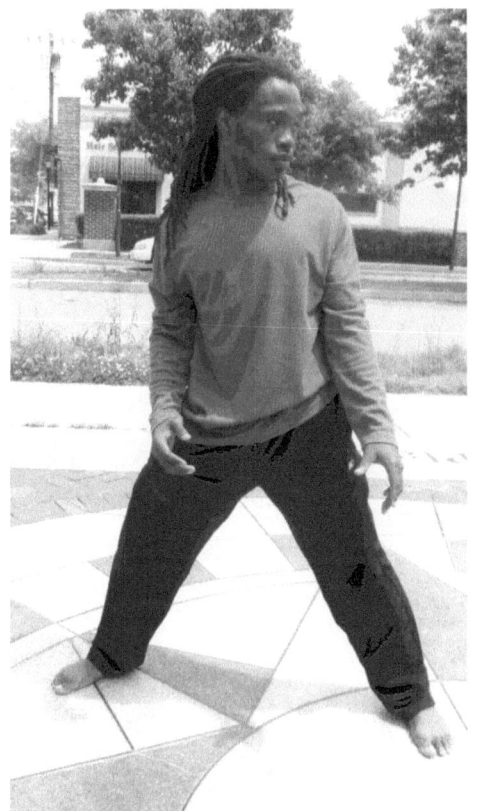

I✳. T✝✝9ひ♭ ⊃Є९ひℨ⨯

17. HAARUB GA'YUSHT

FIGHTING STANCE

Take left fighting stance with your hands down because your next move will be low to the ground.

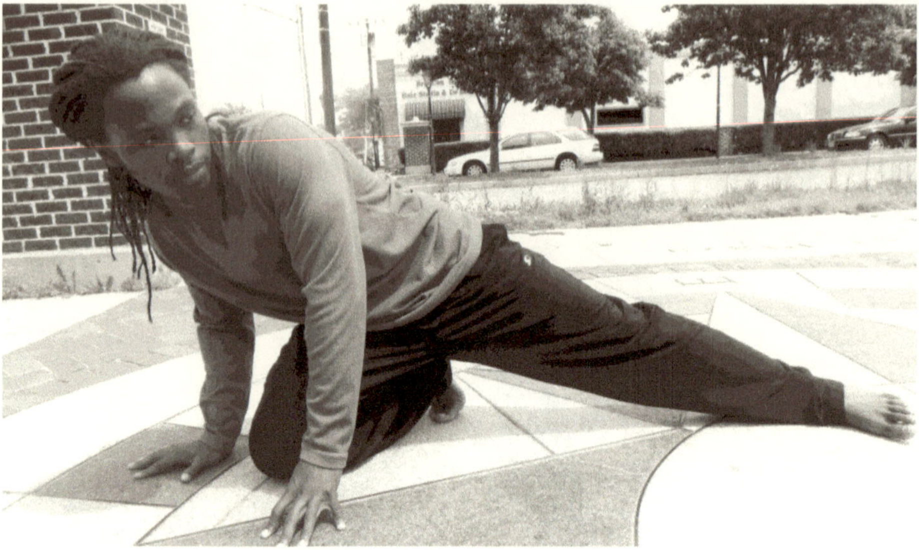

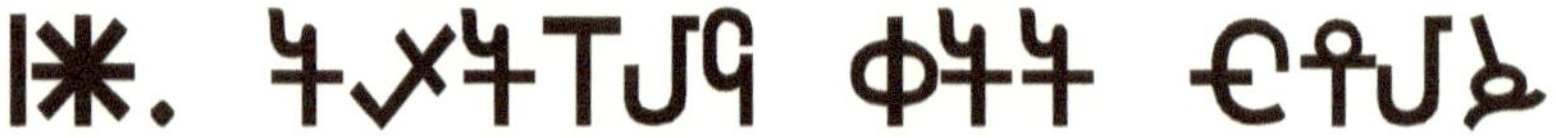

18. ATAHUR PAA A'YUB

WAITING FOR THE ENEMY

Bring your hands and your right knee to the ground. Extend your left leg. Look in the direction of your extended leg.

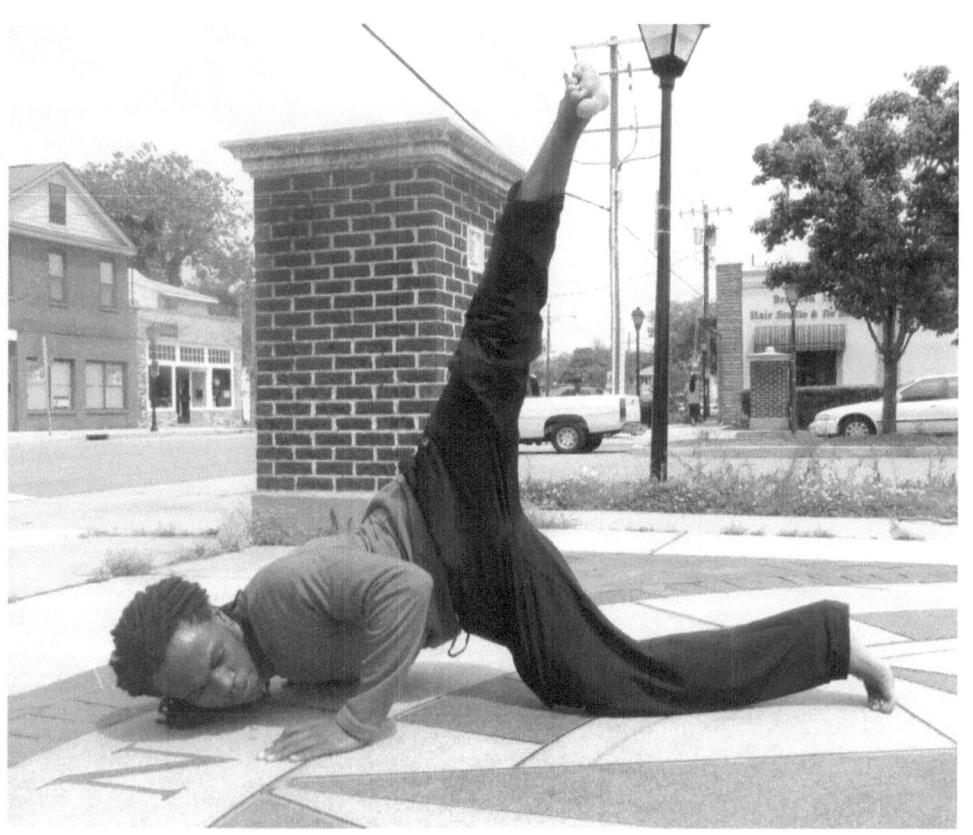

I⊛. ⏀⼡⼡ √Ⴤ⋃√ ੧⼡ḿ⋃Ⴤ

19. PAA LEUL RAFUS

SKY KICK

Bringing your face to the ground, chamber your left leg and kick straight up to the sky. Point the edge of your left foot like a knife.

The First Dance

19 WAYS TO BE DIVINIE

By Baba Afrika

1. Cleanliness Is Next To Godliness.

2. Stay At Peace And Relax.

3. Don't Worry About What Other People Think About You, Worry About What You Think About Yourself.

4. Don't Change, We All Make Mistakes.

5. Block Out All Foreign Thoughts, Just Relax.

6. You Don't Have To Go Along With The Majority.

7. Admit What You Like To Yourself And Others.

8. Accept The Ways The Evil One Distracts You.

9. Accept Agreeable And Disagreeable Beings.

10. Admit What You Don't Like To Yourself And Others.

11. Start Looking Inside, Not Outside A Person.

12. Accept What Is Inside Of You And Not What You Look Like On The Outside.

13. Know That You Are Being Tested By The Evil One, And Accept It.

14. When You Are Teaching Someone, Block Out All Distractions.

15. Make Teaching Your Job, Be Very Serious.

16. Make Sure The Student Overstands You.

17. Don't Start What You Can't Finish.

18. Be Sincere, Don't Try To Impress Anyone.

19. Have No Fear Of Anyone Or Anything, Period.

NAFUN TAWUHAAT

I would like to give thanks to the Most High and the Universe for my creation.

Giving thanks to DARUMA BODHIDHARMA for your incredible journey and giving thanks to masters AZATO and ITOSU for teaching GICHIN FUNAKOSHI I would also like to thank master FUNAKOSHI for his student and thanking him CHOJIN MIYAGI for creating the style of karate called GOJO which is what GOJU SHOREI is a direct descendant of.

I would also like to thank my grandfather sensei Harold Scorpion Burrage for creating the SKS (Scorpion Karate System) and his amazing student my sensei Blade Hillard.

I would like to thank my father Dr. Karaam for leading me to this information and for guiding me my whole life. I would like to thank my mother Monica Garret for giving birth to me so I can accomplish what I must on this physical plane, and my other mother Ryshena Footman for helping to raise me to be a great being and giving thanks to any and all of my friends who were there for me to talk to and comforted me when it was needed.

I would like to thank my siblings :

Akenti, Kayti, Aker, Karum, Safiyyah, Isaiah, Taqee, Quianna

and cousins:

Amunet, Amenti, Asar, Nubi, Sutukh, Farasha, Nekhebet, Ramie, Iyliyya, Wesley and nephews and nieces uncles and aunties just for being there and giving thanks to my grandfathers and grandmothers for raising my parents the way they did so they can raise me properly.

I would like to thank my spiritual teacher Dr. Malachi Z York for the legacy he created and any future ones to come. I would to thank all of my teachers in life younger and older also to thank any of my brothers and sisters who went through a struggle to make the future better us and all of my tribal mothers and fathers. Tawuhaat.....

www.ingramcontent.com/pod-product-compliance
Lightning Source LLC
Chambersburg PA
CBHW050336290526
45785CB00006B/2520